MW00915064

Understanding Cardiomyopathy Heart Diseases

A Comprehensive Guide To The Diagnosis, Treatment, Management And Prevention Of Cardiomyopathy

Doctor Vincent J. Wesley

Copyright © 2023 by Doctor Vincent J. Wesley

All rights reserved. No part of this book may be reproduced, stored in a retrieval system, or transmitted in any form or by any means, electronic, mechanical, photocopying, recording, or otherwise, without the prior written permission of the publisher.

Table Of Contents

Chapter 1: Introduction to Cardiomyopathy

Cardiomyopathy is a group of diseases that affect the heart muscle, most often leading to heart failure and other serious heart problems. It is a life-threatening disorder that demands careful monitoring and control.

Cardiomyopathy may make the heart rigid, enlarged, or thickened and can create scar tissue. As a consequence, the heart can't pump blood adequately to the rest of the body.

With time, the heart grows feeble and cardiomyopathy may lead to heart failure. Therapy may help. But some patients with cardiomyopathy ultimately require a heart transplant.

There are various forms of cardiomyopathy, but all of them entail an anomaly in the size, shape, or structure of the heart muscle. This may lead to the heart being unable to pump blood adequately, which can produce a broad variety of symptoms and consequences.

The most frequent kind is dilated cardiomyopathy, which causes the heart muscle to become stretched out, leading to a diminished capacity to pump blood and an increased risk of heart failure.

Additional forms include hypertrophic cardiomyopathy, which causes the heart muscle to grow thick and inflexible, and restrictive cardiomyopathy, which causes the heart muscle to become stiff and unable to expand adequately.

In certain situations, cardiomyopathy may be caused by an inherited genetic mutation, but it may also be caused by a virus, an autoimmune illness, or certain drugs. Regardless of the cause, cardiomyopathy can be a very serious condition, and it requires careful management to prevent complications and reduce the risk of death.

Therapy may involve lifestyle modifications, medicines, and in rare circumstances, surgery. It is important to recognize the signs and symptoms of cardiomyopathy and seek medical care as soon as possible.

Cardiomyopathy is a serious heart condition that can affect people of all ages. It is crucial to understand the origins, indications and symptoms, and treatment choices to allow in making educated decisions about your health.

With the correct treatment and assistance, cardiomyopathy may be treated and the risk of significant consequences can be reduced.

Thank you for taking the time to learn more about cardiomyopathy.

Chapter 2: Types of Cardiomyopathy

Cardiomyopathy is a disorder of the heart muscle that changes the structure and function of the heart. It may be caused by a multitude of reasons, such as genetic alterations, viral infections, alcohol, and drug misuse.

The most prevalent kinds of cardiomyopathy are:

- Dilated Cardiomyopathy (DCM),

- Hypertrophic Cardiomyopathy (HCM),

- Arrhythmogenic Right Ventricular Dysplasia (ARVD),

- Restrictive Cardiomyopathy (RCM),

- Transthyretin Amyloid Cardiomyopathy (ATTR-CM).

So, let's investigate the different kinds in detail:

1. Dilated Cardiomyopathy (DCM): The most prevalent kind of cardiomyopathy, DCM includes the expansion and thinning of the left ventricle.

The heart's blood-pumping chambers expand (dilate). As a consequence, the heart is unable to pump enough blood throughout the body, resulting in symptoms such as weariness, fluid retention, and shortness of breath.

Dilated Cardiomyopathy (DCM) is a relatively prevalent condition that damages the heart muscle. It is characterized by an enlarged left ventricle, which is unable to contract properly, leading to diminished blood flow.

DCM is a prominent cause of heart failure and is the most prevalent cause of end-stage heart failure in the United States.

DCM happens when the heart muscle gets so feeble that it cannot pump blood adequately. This leads to a reduction in cardiac output and an increase in heart size. With time, the heart becomes too weak to pump blood adequately and the chambers of the heart get enlarged. This causes symptoms such as weariness, shortness of breath, and fluid retention.

DCM may be caused by several reasons, including genetic abnormalities, viral infections, and certain drugs. Additional factors may include excessive blood pressure, coronary artery disease, and diabetes. In other circumstances, the reason may be unknown.

There is no cure for DCM, however, medication may help relieve symptoms and reduce the course of the illness.

Therapy may include drugs to alleviate symptoms, lifestyle adjustments to lower the risk of problems, and cardiac resynchronization treatment (CRT) to enhance the function of the heart. Surgery may also be required in certain circumstances.

DCM is a dangerous illness that may lead to substantial impairment, heart failure, and even death. Early diagnosis and good treatment may help improve symptoms and decrease the risk of complications.

2. Hypertrophic Cardiomyopathy (HCM): HCM is defined by the thickening of the heart muscle, which may lead to restriction of the blood flow and the creation of blood clots. The cardiac muscle thickens.

Symptoms of HCM include; chest discomfort, shortness of breath, dizziness, and palpitations.

HCM is most usually caused by genetic alterations and is the most prevalent cause of sudden cardiac mortality in young athletes.

Hypertrophic Cardiomyopathy (HCM) is a kind of cardiomyopathy, a broad term for a collection of illnesses affecting the heart muscle. It is a hereditary condition that affects the heart muscle, causing it to thicken, and making it difficult for the heart to pump blood. It is a hereditary condition, and also the most frequent kind of cardiomyopathy.

HCM occurs as the heart muscle thickens, making it difficult for the heart to pump blood. This thickening may obstruct the flow of blood through the heart, resulting in a variety of symptoms, including shortness of breath, chest discomfort, and exhaustion. In certain situations, it may also lead to arrhythmia, a condition in which the heart beats too fast or too slow.

The etiology of HCM is not entirely known, however, it is assumed to be linked to a mutation in one or more genes that impact the heart muscle. It is generally caused by a deficiency in the genes that govern the proteins that build up the heart muscle.

HCM is generally diagnosed by physical examination, an electrocardiogram (ECG), echocardiography, and genetic testing. Therapy for HCM comprises drugs to minimize the thickness of the heart muscle, lower the risk of arrhythmia, and reduce the risk of sudden cardiac death.

In certain circumstances, an implanted cardioverter-defibrillator (ICD) may be used to assist regulate arrhythmia. Surgery may also be indicated to lessen the thickness of the heart muscle or to repair the heart valve.

In most instances, HCM may be treated with lifestyle adjustments, such as exercising frequently and consuming a nutritious diet. It is necessary to follow up with a medical practitioner periodically to check the condition. With frequent monitoring, HCM may be controlled efficiently and the risk of problems can be minimized.

3. Restrictive Cardiomyopathy (RCM): RCM is characterized by stiffness of the heart muscle, which limits its ability to fill with blood. This leads to reduced blood flow to the body, resulting in symptoms such as weariness, shortness of breath, and edema of the extremities.

RCM is commonly caused by disorders affecting the heart muscle, such as amyloidosis or sarcoidosis.

Restrictive Cardiomyopathy (RCM) is an uncommon kind of heart muscle disease that inhibits the heart's capacity to adequately fill with blood. It is caused by an abnormal thickening of the heart muscle, which makes it more rigid and inhibits its capacity to relax and fill with blood. This leads to a rise in pressure in the heart and in the lungs, leading to difficulties breathing and weariness.

RCM is a primary cardiomyopathy, meaning that it is not caused by another illness or condition. It is also regarded to be one of the more uncommon kinds of cardiomyopathy, with an estimated frequency of 1 in 10,000 persons.

The most frequent indications and symptoms of RCM are shortness of breath, exhaustion, chest discomfort, palpitations, disorientation, and swelling of the legs and feet.

Diagnosis is often achieved with a combination of physical tests, electrocardiogram (ECG) testing, echocardiography, and a cardiac MRI. Therapy generally includes drugs to alleviate symptoms and enhance heart function, as well as lifestyle adjustments.

In certain circumstances, surgery may be recommended to alleviate pressure in the heart and lungs. This might involve the removal of the pericardium, a thin sac that surrounds the heart, or a cardiac ablation to block aberrant electrical impulses that can induce arrhythmias. In extreme circumstances, a heart transplant may be indicated.

The prognosis for RCM is typically excellent, as long as it is discovered and treated early. With adequate medical treatment, individuals with RCM may live a normal life and even participate in moderate physical activity. Nonetheless, the condition may worsen if left untreated, thus it is crucial to seek medical assistance as soon as possible if there is a discovery of any of the symptoms.

4. Arrhythmogenic Right Ventricular Dysplasia (ARVD): ARVD is defined as the replacement of heart muscle by scar tissue, which may interfere with the normal electrical impulses of the heart and lead to arrhythmias. Diseases in the heart muscle generates abnormal heartbeats.

Symptoms of ARVD include palpitations, dizziness, and fainting. ARVD is most usually caused by genetic mutations.

Arrhythmogenic Right Ventricular Dysplasia (ARVD) is an uncommon kind of cardiomyopathy that affects the right ventricle of the heart. It is a progressive, genetic disorder that is marked by abnormal cardiac rhythms (arrhythmias) and anatomical abnormalities in the right ventricle. ARVD is the main cause of sudden cardiac death (SCD) in young people and is the most prevalent cause of SCD among athletes.

The actual etiology of ARVD is not understood, however, it is considered to have a hereditary component. Mutations in numerous genes have been discovered as possible risk factors for ARVD, including desmoplakin, plakophilin-2, and desmoglein-2. In addition, environmental variables, including smoking and excessive alcohol intake, may raise the risk of ARVD.

The most prevalent symptom of ARVD is palpitations, which are generally perceived as a racing or pounding heart. Additional symptoms might include chest discomfort, shortness of breath, dizziness, fainting, and exhaustion.

An electrocardiogram (ECG) is frequently used to diagnose ARVD since it might reveal signs of arrhythmias and structural alterations in the heart. In certain circumstances, further tests such as echocardiography, cardiac MRI, or cardiac catheterization may be required to confirm the diagnosis.

Treatment of ARVD often comprises drugs to manage the arrhythmias, and lifestyle adjustments to limit the risk of future problems. These adjustments may include avoiding stimulants such as coffee and nicotine and lowering stress. In certain circumstances, an implanted cardioverter-defibrillator (ICD) may be prescribed to manage life-threatening arrhythmias. In extreme circumstances, a heart transplant may be indicated.

ARVD is a severe illness that may have life-threatening effects if not controlled appropriately. It is vital to seek medical assistance in the detection of any of the symptoms linked with ARVD and to follow up on the doctor's recommendations for medication and lifestyle adjustments.

5. Transthyretin Amyloid Cardiomyopathy (ATTR-CM): This is the abnormal protein accumulation (ATTR amyloidosis) in the heart's left ventricle which is the principal blood-pumping chamber.

Transthyretin (TTR) amyloid cardiomyopathy (ATTR-CM) is a rare and lethal type of cardiomyopathy caused by the deposition of misfolded transthyretin (TTR) protein in the heart muscle. This protein deposition may lead to increased heart dysfunction and finally death.

ATTR-CM is a genetic condition caused by mutations in the TTR gene, which is located on chromosome 18. The mutations lead to the creation of aberrant TTR proteins, which are prone to misfolding and produce amyloid deposits in the heart and other organs. These deposits are formed of amyloid fibrils, which are insoluble proteins that collect in the heart and may cause damage to the heart muscle.

The most frequent symptoms of ATTR-CM are shortness of breath, weariness, edema in the legs, and irregular heartbeat. These symptoms may develop over time, leading to heart failure and death.

The diagnosis of ATTR-CM is based on clinical history, physical examination, imaging investigations, and genetic testing. Treatment options include drugs to lessen symptoms, lifestyle modifications, and surgery. In certain circumstances, heart transplantation may be considered to enhance heart function.

ATTR-CM is a progressive illness that may lead to mortality, thus early diagnosis and treatment are critical. Persons with a family history of ATTR-CM must be checked for the disorder since it is heritable. With early diagnosis and treatment, the prognosis for ATTR-CM can be improved.

Note:
Some more sorts of Cardiomyopathy diseases do not fall into these main categories.

Some of them the Include:

I. Broken heart syndrome also known as stress-induced or takotsubo cardiomyopathy, a transient heart enlargement.

II. Chemotherapy-induced cardiomyopathy, a cardiac injury connected to cancer treatment.

IV. Peripartum cardiomyopathy, a kind of Congestive heart failure that develops during or after pregnancy.

Remember that, all kinds of cardiomyopathy may be controlled with lifestyle changes, such as stopping smoking and decreasing alcohol use, and occasionally with drugs or surgical procedures. It is vital to get medical assistance in the cases of symptoms linked with cardiomyopathy, since it may be a life-threatening illness if left untreated.

Chapter 3: Causes of Cardiomyopathy

Cardiomyopathy is a word used to describe a range of disorders that damage the heart muscle. It is a generic phrase used to describe any illness or ailment that affects the heart muscle. It may lead to cardiac failure, arrhythmias, and other problems.

The causes of cardiomyopathy may be split into two categories: main and secondary.

Primary cardiomyopathy is caused by a genetic mutation or an inherited disease. This kind of cardiomyopathy may be noticed in family members since it is handed on from generation to generation.

Primary cardiomyopathy is most usually caused by mutations in genes that are involved in the creation of the heart muscle. These genes may be responsible for directing how the heart contracts and relaxes, or for creating proteins that are involved in the structure of the heart muscle.

Secondary cardiomyopathy is caused by an underlying ailment that damages the heart muscle. This form of cardiomyopathy may be caused by excessive blood pressure, valve dysfunction, infections, alcohol or drug use, or even malignancy. It may also be induced by a toxic response to certain drugs, radiation therapy, or other therapies. In certain circumstances, cardiomyopathy may be caused by a virus or bacterium.

Regardless of the cause, cardiomyopathy may lead to major problems and even death if left untreated. Consequently, it is crucial to get medical assistance as soon as possible if you feel you may have cardiomyopathy. Early identification and treatment may help minimize the risk of problems and improve the quality of life for people afflicted.

In conclusion, primary cardiomyopathy is caused by a genetic mutation or an inherited ailment, whereas secondary cardiomyopathy is caused by an underlying condition that damages the heart muscle. It is vital to get medical assistance on detection of cardiomyopathy, since early diagnosis and treatment may lessen the risk of consequences.

Congenital Cardiomyopathy (CCM)

Congenital cardiomyopathy (CCM) is an uncommon but deadly type of cardiomyopathy, a disease of the heart muscle. It inhibits the heart's capacity to pump blood adequately, resulting in heart failure or other life-threatening consequences. CCM is normally present from birth, however, it may also develop later in life.

CCM may be caused by a variety of genetic abnormalities. These mutations impact the structure and function of the heart muscle and may cause the heart to grow enlarged, weaken, or acquire irregular rhythms.

Symptoms of CCM might include chest discomfort, shortness of breath, weariness, palpitations, and swelling of the feet and ankles.

In certain circumstances, CCM may be treated with drugs, lifestyle modifications, or surgery.

Medicines used to treat CCM include ACE inhibitors, beta-blockers, diuretics, and anticoagulants. Lifestyle adjustments such as avoiding smoking, keeping a healthy weight, and exercising frequently may also assist to improve symptoms of CCM.

Surgery is occasionally done to repair or replace damaged valves or to implant a device that helps the heart beat appropriately.

While there is currently no cure for CCM, early identification and treatment may help to reduce symptoms and avoid catastrophic consequences. Individuals with CCM must be checked periodically by doctors to ensure that the treatment plan is successful. In certain circumstances, supportive treatment such as lifestyle adjustments and medicines may be adequate to manage the illness.

In conclusion, Congenital cardiomyopathy is a dangerous kind of cardiomyopathy that may cause substantial health consequences. Early identification and treatment may help to improve symptoms and minimize the risk of long-term problems. While there is no cure for CCM, drugs, lifestyle modifications, and surgery may be utilized to control the illness.

Acquired Cardiomyopathy Acquired cardiomyopathy is a kind of cardiac disease caused by injury to the heart muscle. It is neither hereditary or congenital but rather caused by a multitude of causes.

They include viral infections, alcohol addiction, drug toxicity, certain drugs, radiation treatment, or other systemic disorders. It is the most frequent kind of cardiomyopathy and is responsible for the majority of occurrences of heart failure.

Acquired cardiomyopathy is frequently characterized by a loss in the heart's capacity to pump blood adequately, resulting in symptoms such as shortness of breath, exhaustion, and swelling in the legs and belly. If left untreated, the illness may lead to major problems such as heart failure, arrhythmias, and even death. Early

diagnosis and timely treatment are
necessary for the best potential results.

Therapy for acquired cardiomyopathy
relies on the underlying etiology. In
certain circumstances, lifestyle
adjustments such as quitting smoking and
restricting alcohol use may be enough to
improve symptoms and lengthen life.
Additional treatments may include drugs,
surgery, or implanted devices such as
pacemakers and defibrillators. In certain
situations, a heart transplant may be
required.

While acquired cardiomyopathy is a
severe illness, it may typically be treated
with adequate medication and lifestyle
adjustments. Early identification and
treatment may help improve symptoms
and minimize the risk of complications.

Additional Causes Of Cardiomyopathy

Healthcare experts may classify cardiomyopathy depending on the general cause.

These two categories are:

- Ischemic cardiomyopathy, induced by heart attacks or coronary artery disease (CAD).

- Non-ischemic cardiomyopathy forms unrelated to CAD.

Sometimes, specialists don't know the etiology of cardiomyopathy (idiopathic).

Several causes or diseases may raise the risk of cardiomyopathy, including:

- Autoimmune illnesses, such as connective tissue diseases.

- Diseases that affect the heart, such as high cholesterol disorders, hemochromatosis, or sarcoidosis.

- Family history of heart disease, cardiomyopathy, or sudden cardiac arrest.

- Prior heart attacks.

- Pregnancy.

Chapter 4: Diagnosing And Test For Cardiomyopathy

Diagnosing cardiomyopathy is vital for the treatment and management of the illness.

The first step in diagnosing cardiomyopathy is to acquire a medical history and do a physical exam. During the medical history, the doctor will ask questions about the patient's family history of heart disease, any symptoms they are having, and any drugs they are taking. The physical exam will examine the patient's heart rate, blood pressure, and any symptoms of fluid in the lungs.

The next stage in diagnosing cardiomyopathy is to run a range of tests. These tests may include an electrocardiogram (ECG), echocardiography, chest X-ray, and cardiac MRI. An ECG may identify any abnormalities in the electrical activity of the heart. An echocardiogram utilizes sound waves to generate an image of the heart, which may be used to check for any abnormalities in the heart's structure or function. A chest X-ray may reveal any fluid or enlargement of the heart. A cardiac MRI may offer a thorough view of the heart and its parts to assist detect any structural abnormalities.

The last step in diagnosing cardiomyopathy is to do a cardiac catheterization. This treatment includes inserting a tiny tube into a blood artery in the arm or groin and threading it to the heart. This enables the doctor to assess the pressure in the heart and the flow of blood.

This test may also be used to determine the quantity of oxygen in the blood.

Diagnosing cardiomyopathy is a critical step in controlling the illness. By collecting a medical history and doing a physical exam, running tests, and conducting a heart catheterization, physicians may properly diagnose cardiomyopathy and prescribe the best treatment strategy for the patient.

Test For Cardiomyopathy

A cardiologist provides a complete examination that may involve a variety of diagnostic tests. Some of them include:

Ambulatory monitoring test which employs equipment that measures the heartbeat.

Cardiac CT utilizes X-rays to generate a movie of the blood arteries and heart. Cardiac MRI employs radio waves and magnets to produce pictures of the heart.

Echocardiogram employs sound waves to generate a picture of the blood flow and heartbeat. Electrocardiogram (EKG) captures the heart's electrical activity.

Workout stress tests elevate heart rates in a controlled manner to assess how the heart reacts.

Cardiac catheterization employs a catheter (a thin tube put via a blood artery) to assess the heart's blood flow and pressure.

Myocardial biopsy analyzes a tiny sample of the heart muscle tissue to search for cell alterations.

Chapter 5: Treatments for Cardiomyopathy

Cardiomyopathy is a disorder of the heart muscle that impairs the heart's capacity to pump blood throughout the body. It may lead to heart failure, arrhythmias, and sudden cardiac death. Therapy of cardiomyopathy varies on the kind and severity of the illness.

For persons with non-ischemic cardiomyopathy, the major objective of therapy is to minimize symptoms, delay the course of the illness, and avoid consequences. Therapy may involve lifestyle adjustments, medicines, and, in rare situations, surgery.

Lifestyle adjustments help control cardiomyopathy. They may include limiting salt consumption, keeping a healthy weight, exercising frequently, and avoiding alcohol and cigarettes.

Medicines are commonly used to treat cardiomyopathy. Popular drugs used to treat cardiomyopathy include beta-blockers, ACE inhibitors, angiotensin receptor blockers (ARBs), and diuretics.

Beta-blockers are used to slow the heart rate and lower blood pressure. ACE inhibitors and ARBs assist to expand the blood arteries, while diuretics help to lower the amount of fluid in the body.

Other drugs, such as digoxin and amiodarone, may be used to assist treat arrhythmias associated with cardiomyopathy. Antiarrhythmic medicines, like sotalol, may also be used to treat arrhythmias.

In certain circumstances, surgery may be required to treat cardiomyopathy. For example, implanted cardioverter-defibrillators (ICDs) may be used to avoid sudden cardiac death. Other forms of surgery, such as coronary artery bypass grafting (CABG) and valve replacement, may also be indicated.

In certain situations, a heart transplant may be essential for persons with severe cardiomyopathy. A heart transplant is a significant procedure that replaces a damaged or diseased heart with a healthy donor heart.

The therapy of cardiomyopathy is personalized depending on the kind and severity of the condition. It is crucial to engage with a healthcare team to discover the optimal treatment strategy for the person.

In addition to medical therapy, lifestyle improvements, such as stress management and a good diet, may help to lessen symptoms and enhance the quality of life.

Medications: Medication is one of the most often used therapies for cardiomyopathy, and many different kinds of drugs may be used to assist control the illness.

The kind and dose of medicine used to treat cardiomyopathy varies on the underlying cause of the ailment and the severity of symptoms. Frequently given drugs for cardiomyopathy include angiotensin-converting enzyme (ACE) inhibitors, angiotensin receptor blockers (ARBs), beta-blockers, calcium channel blockers, diuretics, and anticoagulants.

ACE inhibitors are used to control blood pressure and minimize the burden on the heart muscle. ARBs are used to assist relax and broaden the blood arteries, enabling more blood to flow through them and lessening the pressure on the heart.

Beta-blockers are used to lower the heart rate and increase the efficacy of the heart's pumping function. Calcium channel blockers are used to lessen the contractility of the heart muscle and assist reduce the force of the heart's contractions.

Diuretics are used to assist the body get rid of extra fluid, while anticoagulants are used to lower the danger of blood clots.

In addition to drugs, lifestyle adjustments such as stopping smoking, increasing physical exercise, and eating a nutritious diet are also crucial in controlling cardiomyopathy.

Monitoring and regulating stress levels, as well as undergoing frequent check-ups, may also aid in treating the condition. The aims of therapy for cardiomyopathy are to minimize symptoms, avoid complications, and preserve the patient's quality of life. It is vital to consult with a healthcare practitioner to establish the optimal treatment strategy for a unique requirements.

Implantable Devices: Implantable devices are a kind of therapy for cardiomyopathy, a disorder that impairs the function of the heart. Cardiomyopathy is a chronic illness that may lead to heart failure, stroke, and other consequences if not controlled effectively. Implantable devices are one of the numerous therapy options for cardiomyopathy that attempt to enhance the function of the heart and minimize the symptoms of the condition.

Implantable devices may be used to assist in the control of cardiomyopathy by delivering pacing, defibrillation, and resynchronization of the heart.

Heart pacemakers are the most prevalent form of implanted device used to treat cardiomyopathy. These devices are implanted under the skin and transmit electrical impulses to the heart to control its pace and rhythm.

Different kinds of implantation devices such as implantable cardioverter-defibrillators (ICDs) may be used to send shocks to the heart to restore its normal rhythm. Implantable devices may also be utilized to assist alleviate the symptoms of cardiomyopathy.

Implantable devices such as left ventricular assist devices (LVADs) and implanted hemodynamic devices (IHDs) may be used to help pump blood to the body when the heart is unable to do so. These devices are used to assist alleviate the symptoms of cardiomyopathy such as shortness of breath and exhaustion.

Implantable devices may be a very successful therapy option for cardiomyopathy. These may assist enhance the function of the heart and minimize the symptoms of the condition.

Nevertheless, these gadgets might come with specific hazards such as infection, hemorrhage, and device failure. It is crucial to consider the advantages and hazards of implanted devices with a doctor before choosing treatment.

Overall, implanted devices are a method of therapy for cardiomyopathy that may give excellent symptom alleviation and better cardiac function.

Surgery: Cardiomyopathy is a chronic and gradual degeneration of the heart muscle that may lead to major problems.

Surgery is a method of therapy that may be used to treat cardiomyopathy in some instances. Surgery is performed to repair or replace damaged cardiac tissue, stabilize the structure of the heart, enhance blood flow, and minimize the risk of subsequent issues.

Surgery may be used to treat cardiomyopathy in a variety of ways. It may be used to repair or replace damaged cardiac tissue. This may be done by mending the damaged heart valves, replacing them with artificial valves, or repairing any other damaged parts of the heart. Surgery may also be performed to stabilize the structure of the heart. This may be done by putting a patch over a weakening wall of the heart, or by creating an incision in the wall to build a stronger support system. Surgery may also be performed to enhance blood flow. This may be done by opening up clogged blood arteries or by lowering the size of an enlarged heart chamber.

Surgery may also be done to lessen the risk of additional problems. This may be done by implanting a pacemaker or defibrillator to control the heart's rhythm, or by implanting a device to monitor the heart's electrical activity. In certain circumstances, surgery may be done to remove scar tissue or to implant a device that helps to lower the burden of the heart.

Surgery is not suggested for everyone with cardiomyopathy, and the choice to undergo surgery should be made in cooperation with the healthcare team. The healthcare team will assess the general health, the severity of the cardiomyopathy, and the possible risks and advantages of surgery before making a choice.

Surgery is a serious treatment and comes with it the potential for complications, so it is vital to make sure to understand the risks and benefits before making a choice.

Overall, surgery is a method of therapy that may be utilized to treat cardiomyopathy in specific instances. It may be used to repair or replace damaged cardiac tissue, stabilize the structure of the heart, increase blood flow, and lower the risk of additional issues. But, it is vital to make sure of understanding the risks and advantages of surgery before making a choice and making sure the procedures is been discussed by a healthcare team.

Note that, there is no cure for cardiomyopathy. Nonetheless, the illness can be managed and its growth limited.

Individuals who adopt good lifestyle choices and seek medical care may enjoy a great quality of life with cardiomyopathy.

Chapter 6: Living with Cardiomyopathy

Living with cardiomyopathy may be tough since it is a severe cardiac ailment that can have a substantial effect on a person's quality of life and can even be life-threatening. It is crucial to take the required actions to manage the disease and to recognize the possible hazards linked with it.

The first step in controlling cardiomyopathy is to understand its various forms. There are four primary types: dilated cardiomyopathy (DCM), hypertrophic cardiomyopathy (HCM), restrictive cardiomyopathy (RCM), and arrhythmogenic right ventricular cardiomyopathy (ARVC) (ARVC). Each of these categories has its own set of symptoms, hazards, and therapies.

After a kind of cardiomyopathy is recognized, it is crucial to work with a doctor to design a treatment plan that is specific to the individual. Therapy may involve lifestyle adjustments such as a low-sodium diet, frequent exercise, and stopping smoking, as well as drugs to alleviate symptoms and treat the heart problem, such as angiotensin-converting enzyme (ACE) inhibitors or beta blockers.

In certain circumstances, a pacemaker or an implanted cardioverter-defibrillator (ICD) may be required.

It is also crucial to recognize the possible hazards linked with cardiomyopathy and to be aware of any warning symptoms.

Symptoms may include chest discomfort, shortness of breath, irregular heartbeats, lightheadedness, and fainting. If any of these symptoms arise, it is crucial to seek medical assistance immediately once.

Living with cardiomyopathy may be tough, but with the correct treatment plan and lifestyle improvements, it is possible to manage the illness and lessen the dangers associated with it. It is crucial to be proactive and work closely with a doctor to design a strategy that will assist keep the illness under control.

Lastly, it is crucial to remember that there is no cure for cardiomyopathy, thus it is necessary to take efforts to control the illness and to keep updated about the newest breakthroughs in therapy. With the correct care and support, it is possible to live well and retain a decent quality of life.

Signs Of Cardiomyopathy?

Some people have no cardiomyopathy symptoms. As the condition advances, others may experience:

- Fatigue,

- Heart palpitations (rapid heartbeat),

- Shortness of breath (dyspnea),

- Syncope (fainting).

How Does Cardiomyopathy Impact The Body?

When cardiomyopathy progresses, the development of additional cardiac disorders may arise such as:

- Arrhythmias (irregular heartbeats),

- Heart failure,

- Heart valve disorders, including heart valve disease, and so on....

Chapter 7: Prognosis of Cardiomyopathy

Cardiomyopathy is a form of cardiac disease that affects the structure and function of the heart muscle. It is a potentially life-threatening disorder that may lead to cardiac failure, arrhythmia, and other consequences. Depending on the kind of cardiomyopathy and the severity of the illness, the prognosis might vary.

In general, the prognosis for cardiomyopathy is favorable if the illness is discovered and treated early. If the problem is discovered and therapy is begun early, it is feasible for the patient to return to a regular lifestyle with no long-term repercussions. Nevertheless, if the illness is not recognized and treated early, the prognosis is far less good.

The prognosis of cardiomyopathy also relies on the kind of cardiomyopathy. Dilated cardiomyopathy is the most frequent kind and is generally caused by an underlying ailment such as a virus or autoimmune disease. The prognosis for this form of cardiomyopathy is typically favorable, as long as the underlying condition is cured and the patient gets adequate medical treatment. Hypertrophic cardiomyopathy is a more severe type of cardiomyopathy that may lead to major consequences such as heart failure.

The prognosis for this form of cardiomyopathy is less favorable, however, it is feasible to treat the illness with drugs and lifestyle adjustments.

Restrictive cardiomyopathy is an uncommon kind of cardiomyopathy that may be difficult to identify and cure. The prognosis for this kind of cardiomyopathy is quite bad, and the patient may need a heart transplant to live.

Generally, the prognosis for cardiomyopathy varies on the kind of illness, the underlying cause, and the severity of the ailment. Early diagnosis and treatment may considerably improve the prognosis, whereas delaying diagnosis and treatment might have catastrophic repercussions. It is vital to seek medical assistance as soon as any signs of cardiomyopathy are discovered to achieve the best potential result.

How Common Is Cardiomyopathy?

Cardiomyopathy may affect anybody of any age or ethnicity. Around 1 in 500 individuals have cardiomyopathy.

Certain kinds of cardiomyopathy are more likely in some persons than in others. For example, dilated cardiomyopathy is more frequent among African individuals.

Dilated and arrhythmogenic cardiomyopathy are more frequent in men.

How Does Cardiomyopathy Affect Children And Teenagers?

Pediatric cardiomyopathy may afflict children and teens of any gender, ethnicity, or age. It is more likely to develop in babies than in older children.

Children may inherit cardiomyopathy. Very infrequently, they may develop cardiomyopathy from a viral infection. Around 75% of the time, healthcare practitioners don't know what causes the disease.

Some children may have no cardiomyopathy symptoms until they have sudden heart arrest. Yet, early discovery and treatment may enhance a child's prognosis.

Children with a cardiomyopathy diagnosis require regular treatment with a cardiologist (heart specialist). They will need daily medicine. Depending on the etiology, kind, and stage of cardiomyopathy, many adolescents and teens may live with little lifestyle constraints.

Chapter 8: Prevention of Cardiomyopathy

Cardiomyopathy is a disorder in which the heart muscle becomes weaker, enlarged, and/or rigid, making it difficult for the heart to pump blood adequately. It may lead to cardiac failure or arrhythmias. Prevention of cardiomyopathy entails lifestyle adjustments such as keeping a healthy weight, eating a heart-healthy diet, avoiding cigarettes and alcohol, and exercising frequently.

Keeping a healthy weight is vital to avoid cardiomyopathy. This entails consuming a diet rich in fruits, vegetables, whole grains, and lean meats while reducing processed and fried foods.

Consuming a heart-healthy diet may also help minimize the risk of cardiomyopathy. This involves ingesting enough fruits, vegetables, healthy grains, and lean proteins while reducing saturated fat, trans fat, and salt.

Avoiding smoke and alcohol is also crucial for cardiomyopathy prevention. Smoking may damage the heart and raise the risk of cardiomyopathy. Alcohol use should be minimized since it might weaken the heart muscle and elevate blood pressure.

Exercising consistently is also beneficial for avoiding cardiomyopathy. Frequent physical exercise may help maintain a healthy weight and improve the heart. It may also help relieve stress and enhance general wellness.

In addition, it is vital to practice stress management strategies such as yoga, meditation, and deep breathing exercises. Stress may raise the risk of cardiomyopathy and other heart problems.

Lastly, it is crucial to obtain frequent check-ups with the doctor. The doctor can monitor the heart health and take preventative actions to lower the chances of cardiomyopathy. A doctor may also help build a strategy to control any current risk factors for cardiomyopathy.

In summary, prevention of cardiomyopathy entails lifestyle adjustments like keeping a healthy weight, eating a heart-healthy diet, avoiding nicotine and alcohol, exercising frequently, adopting stress management strategies, and obtaining regular check-ups with your doctor. These actions may help lower the risk of cardiomyopathy and enhance overall heart health.

How Can I Lower The Risk Factors Of Cardiomyopathy?

There is no method to avoid congenital (inherited) kinds of cardiomyopathy. Various actions may be performed to lessen the risk of diseases that might develop cardiomyopathy.

Some of these stages include:

- Controlling your blood pressure,

- Maintaining your cholesterol within safe values,

- Treating underlying diseases such as sleep apnea or diabetes,

- Arranging frequent visits with a healthcare practitioner,

- Taking all meds as recommended.

Conclusion

In conclusion, cardiomyopathy is a significant cardiac disorder that affects the structure and function of the heart muscle. It may be caused by a multitude of circumstances, including hereditary or acquired disorders, or even particular drugs or poisons.

Symptoms may include chest discomfort, shortness of breath, exhaustion, and irregular heartbeats. Treatment options vary depending on the kind and severity of the problem and may include drugs, lifestyle modifications, and in rare circumstances, surgery.

It is crucial to get medical assistance on detection of symptoms linked with cardiomyopathy. Early detection and action may help lessen the likelihood of additional problems.

Overall, cardiomyopathy is a severe ailment that may have catastrophic repercussions if left untreated. It is vital to adopt preventative steps, including regular exercise, good nutrition, and avoiding certain drugs, to help lower the chance of acquiring this illness.

With prompt intervention, cardiomyopathy may be treated and controlled, enabling people afflicted to continue a healthy, productive life.

Made in the USA
Monee, IL
12 January 2024

51638950R00039